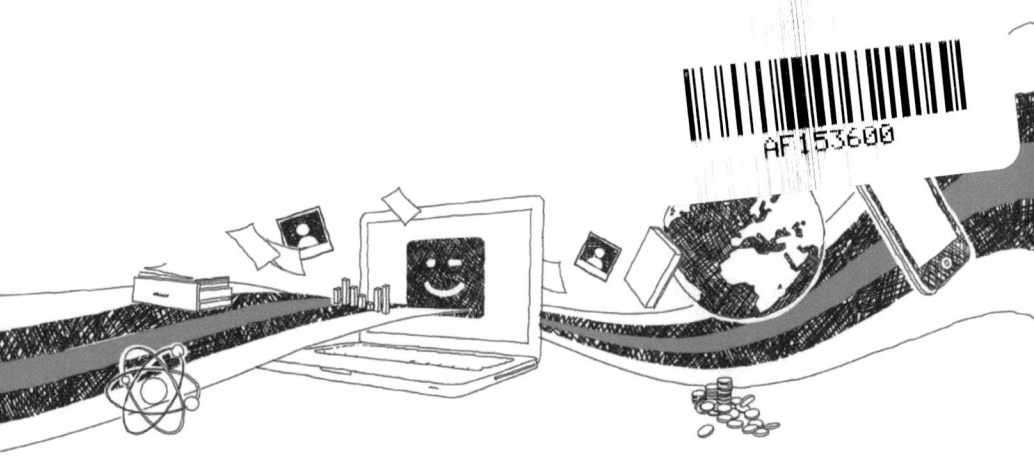
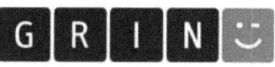

Talent management in short track speed skating

Emil Imre

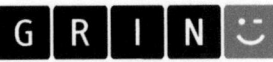

Bibliographic information published by the German National Library:

The German National Library lists this publication in the National Bibliography; detailed bibliographic data are available on the Internet at http://dnb.dnb.de.

ISBN: 9783389127070
This book is also available as an ebook.

© GRIN Publishing GmbH
Trappentreustraße 1
80339 München

Print and binding: Books on Demand GmbH, Norderstedt, Germany
Printed on acid-free paper from responsible sources.

The present work has been carefully prepared. Nevertheless, authors and publishers do not incur liability for the correctness of information, notes, links and advice as well as any printing errors.

GRIN web shop: https://www.grin.com/document/1574319

Talent management in short track speed skating

Table of contents

1. Introduction

Talent management has been a preoccupation of societies for thousands of years, and ancient Greece was no exception. Throughout history, all societies have sought to identify and develop individuals with outstanding abilities. However, the concept of talent has evolved over time and the methods of talent management have constantly evolved. Although everyone intuitively knows what we are talking about when we talk about talent, its precise definition is still debated by philosophers, educators and psychologists. Talent is not simply a single ability, but a complex set of qualities that develops as a result of a combination of factors. Generally speaking, talent is a potential that enables an individual to excel in some area. Several theories have attempted to explain the development and functioning of talent, one of the best known being Renzulli's (1978) three-part model, which posits that talent consists of three components: above-average ability, creativity and commitment to a task. Its concept is also a central issue in the world of sport, as outstanding and successful athletes are often perceived as possessing some special and intangible ability that distinguishes them from the average. Outstanding performance in sport often depends not only on innate talent, but also on the effectiveness of talent management and the quality of development support programmes (Baker et al., 2017; Grainger et al., 2024). Talent management is a systematic and thoughtful process that aims to develop young athletes with individual abilities to the highest possible level of performance (Baker et al, 2017; Vaeyens et al., 2008; Telegdi et al., 2024). Short track speed skating is an exceptionally complex and demanding sport in which athletes are required to achieve maximum performance in an extremely short time, a very complex sport both technically and physically, in which speed, flexibility and tactical awareness are equally important (Konings et al, 2015; Kuper & Sterken, 2003; Morrison et al., 2005). In these races, athletes cover the distance in just 1-2 minutes, so concentration and quick reactions are of paramount importance, as a single small mistake can determine the outcome (Konings et al., 2015)Short track speed skaters compete in special conditions: not only speed and technical preparation are required, but also the ability to concentrate properly in a cold environment on ice. The cold is a challenge in itself, as it can affect the athlete's physical and mental performance, especially when short but intense periods of concentration are required during the competition (Morrison et al., 2005). In addition, the individual nature of the sport means that athletes have to rely on their own resources rely on their own resources and do not have the possibility of teamwork or outside help as in team sports (e.g. football).

The aim of the research is to explore what specific talent management methods can help in short track speed skating and how to support the mental preparation of athletes for these special circumstances. Currently, the example of a biofeedback and psychological skill development programme developed for the Canadian short track speed skating team demonstrates the potential for innovation, using an integrated approach to optimise athletes' self-regulation to maximise performance under competition and pressure. These practices include biofeedback techniques to promote conscious control of bodily responses through psychology, which have already been successfully applied in Canada in preparation for the 2010 Vancouver Olympics. Our central research question is also what factors play a key role in talent management in a sport that requires intense concentration and physical exertion in a very short period of time. The novelty of this thesis lies in the fact that it light on sport-specific challenges that are primarily specific to individual sports that take place in a cold environment for short periods time. In this way, the findings can contribute to the field of sport science that adapts the application of talent management methods to the specific requirements of a sport. Our central research question is what factors play a key role in talent management in a sport requiring intense concentration and physical exertion over a very short period of time, and more specifically, how consistent are the players in the sport with regard to the requirements of the sport, especially in the area of mental ability.

1.1. Literature review: mental challenges in short track speed skating

This chapter will focus on the mental and technical challenges of short track speed skating, focusing on the importance of mental challenges for athletes, coaches, sports psychologists and parents. Short track speed skating, in which athletes compete on relatively small tracks at high speeds, has specific physical and mental challenges. This sport requires intense concentration, as competitors have to constantly make decisions about accelerating at the right time, turning techniques and avoiding competitors. In a performance that is short in duration but requires maximum effort, athletes must be able to maintain a high level of concentration and technical precision while executing fast, sharp movements (Menting et al., 2019). The sport is also technically challenging, as skaters must be able to perform at a high level of maintain stability while achieving extraordinary accelerations. Lower extremity muscle strength is key to skaters' performance; research by Felser et al. (2015) shows that isometric and concentric muscle strength has a direct impact on skaters' speed and time. Maintaining ankle and knee stabilisation during fast skating is essential, especially as unstable movements are often further complicated by the extra degree of freedom provided by skates. The cold environment poses a significant challenge for short track speed skaters as low temperatures affect muscle performance and maintenance of body temperature, which also directly affects mental state (Gatterer et al, 2021)Slowing muscle function and neuromuscular responses in cold conditions reduces reaction time and concentration, which are critical factors for quick decisions and movements in short and intense competitions (Castellani & Young, 2016; Cheung et al., 2016). In addition, mental stress caused by cold environments increases psychological strain, which can interfere with athletes' ability to focus. According to Beauchamp et al. (2012), the Canadian Olympic team's biofeedback and mental skill development programs help athletes manage this stress more effectively. Research emphasizes that it is critical for athletes to warm up properly, dress appropriately, and adapt to the cold to optimize their performance and reduce the negative effects of the cold (Gatterer et al., 2021)." Mental challenges include short periods of intense concentration, which is essential for success. According to McMorris and Rayment (2007), short, intense physical workloads can significantly affect sport skills that require perceptual and motor decisions. Their results suggest that high-intensity, short-duration exercises negatively affect athletes' performance in these types of tasks, which are also required in speed skating. For coaches, mental challenges include the need to adapt competition strategies quickly and to monitor athletes' mental state continuously. According to Grant (2006), coaches need to be versatile and sensitive enough to immediately recognise mental changes in athletes and intervene quickly when necessary to maintain or restore their athletes' mental focus and motivation. Comprehensive coaching psychology approaches, discussed by Grant and Palmer (2015), highlight the importance of integrating positive psychological elements that can help coaches to create a more supportive and goal-oriented environment. In addition, Griffo et al's (2019) review of sport coaching highlights the need for coaches to systematically apply the latest scientific knowledge and methods in their coaching practice to effectively address the mental and physical needs of athletes to ensure peak performance is achieved and maintained. For parents mental challenges are mainly related to emotional support during competitions and maintaining their child's commitment to sport. It is important for parents to be able to contribute positively to their children's mental wellbeing, especially in coping with setbacks and pressure, which can have a significant impact on young athletes' performance and passion for sport. According to Knight et al (2017), parental support plays a crucial role in the psychosocial development of athletes and is particularly important during competitive periods when children may experience stress and pressure. According to Burke and colleagues (2021), parent education programs that target positive parental support can improve interactions between parents and children, reducing stress and increasing enjoyment and self-confidence in athletes. Sports psychologists play an important role in the mental preparation of speed skaters, particularly in addressing pre-competition anxiety, increasing mental resilience and teaching techniques such as visualisation and biofeedback. These techniques help athletes to manage high stress levels during competition. According to Danish and Nellen (1997), sport psychologists can use sport as a tool to develop life skills, especially among at-risk youth, which is directly linked to the mental preparation of athletes. McDougall et al. (2015) emphasize that sport psychologists face a number of challenges in elite sport environments, including managing diverse relationships and continuously monitoring the mental health of athletes. Anderson, Knowles, and Gilbourne (2004) highlight the importance of reflective practice to help sport psychologists better understand and manage the challenges of working with athletes, thus improving athletes' mental preparation and performance in competitions. For athletes, mental challenges include the need for rapid decision-making during competitions, which requires intense mental focus and undistracted concentration. According to Oliver, McCarthy, and Burns (2020), attention is a teachable skill that directly contributes to the ability to concentrate, which is vital during short, intense competitions. Nam, Choi, and Cho's (2022) research emphasizes that athletes' psychological skills, such as stress tolerance and mental resilience, are key in speed skating, where competitors must adapt to rapidly changing circumstances.

According to Wilks (1991), stress management techniques such as relaxation exercises and positive psychological support are essential to improve sports performance and reduce the risk of injury. These techniques help athletes manage the psychological stress during competition, which has a direct impact on physical performance. Visit effective stress management reduces the effects of negative emotions such as anxiety and frustration, which can hinder athletes' ability to make quick and accurate decisions. Mental preparedness, including the development of self-confidence and goal-setting skills, is also essential in short-term, intense sports. As part of their preparation, athletes need to learn how to use mental imagery and biofeedback techniques to help optimise their mental state before and during competition, enhancing performance and reducing mental fatigue (Nam et al, 2022). Research has shown that athletes' mental preparedness, which includes increased stress tolerance and emotional regulation techniques, has a direct influence on sport performance and competitiveness (Nam et al., 2022; Wilks, 1991). Harnessing these mental resources helps athletes maintain focus and agility during competition, which is essential for success.

2. Objective

The aim of the research is to identify the most important factors in talent management in short track speed skating. It is hypothesised **that the players in the sport of short track speed skating are not unified in their understanding of the requirements of the sport, particularly in the area of mental ability.** This issue is of particular relevance to sports science, as a deep understanding of the differences in mental ability between athletes can contribute to the development of more effective training methods and support strategies that better take into account individual differences.

3. Materials and methods

This research uses qualitative methods to investigate the role of talent management in short track speed skating, with a particular focus on the development of young athletes. The main data collection method used in the research is a semi-structured interview, which provides a deeper insight into the talent management processes in short track speed skating, the coaching experiences and the personal experiences of the athletes. This method was chosen to collect data within a consistent framework, while also offering flexibility in the questions to include new themes and ideas that emerge during the interview. This method is particularly advantageous when the phenomena under study are complex and require in-depth understanding, as in this case the talent development processes in short track speed skating. According to Kállay (2008), semi-structured interviews facilitate the elicitation of interviewees' personal experiences, feelings and a detailed exploration of their motivations, which is essential to answer the research questions. Thematic analysis, one of the most common forms of qualitative data analysis, was used to process the data. This involved grouping the collected interview data into categories to identify frequently occurring patterns and themes. In this way, we gained a structured yet in-depth insight into important factors in talent management.

3.1. Sample and sampling procedure

Convenience sampling was used to select the subjects. As described by Boncz (2015), this method relies on the availability of easily accessible subjects. Participants were interviewed by phone or some kind of video communication application and were interviewed for 30-60 minutes, which was influenced by the habitus of the interviewees. The interviews were conducted with eight different actors, all with relevant experience in the field of talent management. The table below presents the interviewees.

coach 1	Men	46 year	He has been a coach for 15 years. He has followed the careers of many talented athletes, many of whom have achieved success in international competitions. This interview aims to give an insight into the methods used to identify and develop talent.
sports psychologist 1	Women	32	He has been working in this for 6 years. She is a sports psychologist specialised in talent management, working specifically with young athletes. The focus of this interview is on the role of mental coaching, with a special focus on concentration and stress management.
Athlete 1	Men	18 annual	18-year-old who has won several medals at the national championships. He was enrolled in a talent programme at an early age and we will explore the factors that contributed to his development through his personal experiences.
Parent 1	Women	46 annual	A parent of a talented athlete who is actively involved in supporting their child's sporting career. The discussion will focus on the role of family background in talent development.
Sports organisational manager	Men	52 annual	Head of a national sports federation's talent management programme, providing insight into the operation of sport structures and talent management programmes, particularly in short track speed skating.
sports psychologist 2	Women	37	8 years of experience in developing the mental skills of young and elite athletes, with a focus on methods to improve stress management and concentration.
Parent 2	Men	49 year	Active participation and support in the child's sporting career, including logistical and emotional support, and coordination of training and competition programmes.
Athlete 2	Women	19 annual	Personal experience of the mental and physical challenges of speed skating, techniques and strategies used in competitions and training

1. Table 1: Presentation of interviewees[1]. Source: own ed.

---

[1] The names and other identifying information of the interviewees will not shared at their request, so we will refer to them only by the codes you see in the table, instead of by their personal names.

4. Results

4.1. Athletes' mental abilities and their development

Developing the mental skills of athletes is a priority in short track speed skating, where quick decision making, high levels of concentration and stress tolerance are essential, all interviewees confirmed. There were many different opinions, but during the interviews, athletes, coaches and psychologists all confirmed that the development of mental skills is the basis for the long-term success of athletes. One athlete, who is 19 years old and has competed in several international competitions, said, *"In the days before competitions, maximising my concentration is the biggest challenge. My psychologist taught me relaxation techniques that have significantly improved my performance."* This confirms the extent to which mental preparation can improve the competitiveness of athletes. One coach, 46 years old and a veteran competitor with decades of experience, says: *"Over the years I have learned that mental toughness often matters more than physical preparedness. I often help younger athletes to recognise how to stay calm and collected under the nervous pressure of competition."* This comment may that developing mental skills has not only immediate but also long-term benefits. The role of coaches in developing mental skills is also paramount. A 32-year-old sports psychologist who works particularly with young talent shared, *"Mental training is as fundamental a part of daily training as physical preparation. We work together to develop programmes to help athletes better manage the psychological pressure of competition."* This suggests the importance of collaboration between different professionals in developing the mental skills of athletes. A comment from a young 18-year-old athlete in particular illustrates the differences between different age groups and levels of competition: *"I feel that mental preparation is often overshadowed in the youngest athletes because we focus on technical development. The first time I was faced with a big competition, I realised that I was not mentally prepared for it and it really affected my performance."* This shows that there can be gaps in mental preparation for athletes at an early stage of their career, which supports the assumption that not all athletes receive the same mental support or training.

In contrast, a more experienced 46-year-old coach says: *"Mental skills development has always been part of my training, because I know that psychological preparedness can be crucial as well as physical strength. I have also introduced specific techniques such as visualisation and positive reinforcement, which have helped me in the most difficult races."* This quote shows that there are coaches who have recognised the importance of developing mental skills early on and have consciously integrated them into their training routines. Although this may have been influenced by the sporting background of the coach, who presumably had already tried to develop these routines on the basis of his experience, as he was aware of the shortcomings of the training programmes of young people. The differences are not only between athletes but also between coaches. The head of the sports organisation, who has decades of experience, said: *"Even as a coach, part of my philosophy was to treat each athlete as an individual and not as an equal. Some need more support on the mental side, while others handle the pressure of competition well on their own."* This clearly shows that coaches approach mental skill development in different ways, taking into account the individual needs and skill levels of each athlete. The experience of the athlete's past may also play a role in this approach. These differences and individual approaches show that the players in the sport of short track speed skating are indeed not uniform in terms of the requirements of the sport, especially in the area of mental skills, everyone is different and preparing them accordingly will lead to greater success. Athletes of different ages, experience levels and personalities respond and require mental support in different ways, supports the hypothesis of our research and highlights the need for tailoring talent management strategies. Based on interviews with athletes, coaches, and psychologists of different gender and experience levels, it is evident that the players in the sport of short track speed skating are not unified in their understanding of the demands and mental challenges of the sport. Female athletes often tend to place more emphasis on mental support and stress management techniques than their male counterparts. The 19-year-old female athlete said, *"Dealing with stress and anxiety before competitions is what I work on most with my psychologist. Female athletes are often under more pressure to perfection and expectations."*

In contrast, male athletes often receive a different type of mental training, which focuses on managing competitiveness and aggression. A 46-year-old male coach shared, *"We teach boys to use the adrenaline of competition to their advantage and to manage it better.*

physical challenges. Although I think this approach is sometimes sexist and counterproductive, as girls are traditionally allowed more emotionality."

Interviews with female psychologists also confirmed that they often take a different approach to the mental training of athletes. A female psychologist who has worked in the sport for almost a decade said, "As *a female psychologist, I see the importance of open communication and the emotional support we provide. In addition, the role of family support is also given more emphasis when I work with female athletes.*"

Based on the data collected during the interviews, it became clear that the differences between athletes, be it in terms of gender, age or experience, require a number of different approaches to mental skills development. These differences and individual needs highlight the key importance of tailoring talent management strategies and the need to into account different demographic and psychological factors when developing the mental skills of athletes. This complex approach will ensure that each athlete receives the necessary support and training tailored to their needs and circumstances, which will contribute to their long-term success in the sport of short track speed skating.

4.2. Coaching strategies and their impact on mental ability

Among the challenges in the sport of short track speed skating, mental skills are a key area, which are developed through coaching strategies. Coaches play a key role in shaping athletes' mental abilities, increasing competitiveness and developing psychological resilience. During the interviews, the participants showed that there are significant differences in training methods and mental strategies used. A 46-year-old coach, who was himself a former competitor, highlighted the following: "*Every athlete is unique and as such, mental training must be personalised. This is especially important for young athletes who are just getting used to the pressure of competition.*"

The sports psychologist, a 32-year-old woman who is also currently working with the junior team, shared how interesting it is when young boys are first exposed to stress management techniques. There is still a common perception that "*boys don't* cry", as she puts it, so *"when we suddenly start dealing with our mental health, it takes them by surprise, many people see it as downright unnecessary or don't understand why it's happening".*

These strategies are particularly important in the period before and during competition, when athletes face their greatest psychological challenges. The 37-year-old sports psychologist says: "*During mental preparation, I work with coaches to coordinate physical and mental training so that athletes can prepare for competitions in a balanced and optimal way.*"

The socio-economic background also has a significant impact on coaching strategies. An experienced coach who has worked with athletes from different backgrounds said, "*Background has a big influence on the mental skills that need to be developed. Athletes from difficult backgrounds often need more emphasis on building confidence and mental toughness.*"

Coaches' strategies address not only individual differences between athletes, but also gender differences. For female athletes, emotional support techniques often predominate, while for men, competitive and results-focused approaches predominate. One female athlete summed up her experience: "*My coach has always put a lot of emphasis on being mentally strong and learning to manage the stress of competition.*" She stressed that she felt that the cooperation between the coach and the sports psychologist had a positive effect on her. Many of his peers have told him about bad experiences when they heard coaches say things like "*don't whine*" and "*don't be pushy*", but he considers himself lucky because he knows that the sports psychologist is more advanced in dealing with emotional issues.

The interviews suggest that coaching strategies and their impact on mental ability are highly variable, and how individual coaches adapt to the individual needs of their athletes. The differences between the players in the sport of short track speed skating are also reflected in their coaching approaches, which supports our hypothesis that the players in the sport are not uniform in their approach to the demands of the sport, particularly in the area of mental skills.

4.3. The role of family and sports organisational support in the development of mental skills

Family support plays a crucial role in developing the mental skills of athletes, especially young talent. The emotional and logistical support provided by families support is essential for the development of athletes. A 19-year-old female *athlete* said. *Knowing they are there for me reduces stress. But it's clear that my mum and dad had a different way of supporting me, there's no question about it. "*

Support from sporting organisations is also key, particularly in providing programmes and resources to develop mental skills. One sports psychologist who works with various teams highlighted, *"Sporting organisations need to ensure they have adequate mental health support, including access to qualified psychologists and mental skills development programmes. "*

The impact of family and sport organisational support on athletes' performance and mental is significant. The head of the sports organisation, who was also interviewed, stressed that the role of sports clubs and associations is as important as that of the family in talent management. *"The role of sports clubs is not only to provide training but also to support athletes' performance in the long term, including mental preparation and access to the necessary resources,"* he explained. He said sports organisations also have a responsibility to provide adequate professional support for athletes, especially when the cost of competitions and training camps is beyond the reach of the family.

The parent also spoke about how the support provided by sports organisations can make life much easier families, but also pointed out that in many cases individual resources are needed. *"Without the support of clubs and associations, we probably wouldn't be able to keep our children in sport at this level, but a lot of the burden still rests on our shoulders. Speed skating requires special equipment, and there are costs that have to be raised somehow before each competition,"* shared the parent.

5. Results and discussion

The results show that the success of the talent management process is closely linked to the balance between the mental and physical preparation of athletes. Research has confirmed that the development of mental skills such as stress management, perseverance, and quick decision making are essential   in maximising the   performance   of athletes.   Training methods highlighted by coaches and sports psychologists include relaxation techniques, visualisation and stress management practices, which the research has shown to contribute directly to competitive performance.

5.1. Comparison of results with research on this topic

An analysis of the specific mental and physical challenges of speed skating shows that, in addition to strong physical skills, the development of mental stamina is essential to maximise athletes' performance. For speed skaters, the need to perform for short periods of time but with maximum concentration creates a unique situation that distinguishes them from athletes in other sports. The cold environment, the individual nature of the competitions and the intensity of the performance focused on a short period of time are factors that require specific mental preparation and endurance (Gatterer et al., 2021; Castellani & Tipton, 2015). According to the interviewees, not only physical training but also individual mental preparation is important in speed skating. The sports psychologist explained that speed skaters regularly use visualisation and relaxation techniques to help them find calmness and prepare for maximum performance before competitions. This approach is also supported by Beauchamp et al (2012), who argue that biofeedback and mental skills development in short track speed skaters helps to manage cold-induced stress and maintain emotional control. Continuing the comparison, the comparison between the long-term athlete preparation model discussed by Telegdi (2021) and the specifications of the sport of short track speed skating provides significant insights. The LTAD (Long-Term Athlete Development) model presented by Telegdi has already proven its usefulness in many sports, and its principles have been adapted by the Hungarian speed skating discipline, significantly improving the preparation of athletes and talent management. According to Telegdi (2021), long-term goals and conscious athlete development programmes can significantly improve athletes' competitive performance and overall well-being. In contrast, the results presented in our research suggest that, although the development of mental skills is key, there are significant differences in levels of preparedness and development opportunities between athletes, supporting our hypothesis that there is a lack of consistency in the development of athletes' mental skills and the ways in which they are developed, which requires further specific interventions. Bognár et al. (2006) emphasise the importance of the role of parents in sports talent management, which is in line with our present research, where we investigated the effects of family support and sport organisational background on athletes' mental abilities. The paper shows that active parental involvement and support is essential for the development of young athletes, especially in terms of mental preparation. Parental support can help athletes to better manage the psychological pressure and stress of competitions, which is in line with our research findings and knowledge in the field of sport psychology. It is noteworthy that a comparison of my research with other studies found in the field draws sharp contours, especially when it comes to a deeper understanding of coaching roles and environmental influences in the sport of speed skating. In his assessment of coaching roles, Telegdi (2023) emphasises the importance of considering the different approaches of coaches in domestic speed skating to understand the differences between the actors in the sport. The diversity of coaching philosophies and methodologies challenges the use of standardised coaching protocols, which can be paralleled with the different mental skill development strategies identified by this research. This highlights how the individual needs of athletes and coaches can vary, which should be taken into account in domestic practice. In their study of environmental factors, Telegdi, Bognár and Géczi (2024) highlight the important role of the environment in the talent development of speed skating. This analysis is closely related to the results of current research, which shows that family and sport organisational support can have a crucial influence on the mental development of athletes. The influence of environmental factors supports the view that the development of athletes' mental skills is not only dependent on coaching interventions, but also on the wider environment, including family background and sport organisational structures. Compared to the literature, it can be argued that mental techniques such as visualization and stress management methods remain the most effective tools for speed skaters, especially due to the cold and the individual nature of competitions (Beauchamp et al., 2012; Gatterer et al., 2021). The results confirm that the cold environment requires not only physical but also mental preparation, which is necessary to maintain concentration and make quick decisions. This research may provide new perspectives for the development of talent management programmes and guidance for coaches and sport organisations to support the development of athletes through targeted mental training.

Overall, the data collected in my research and the parallels between previous studies emphasise that taking into account the individual needs of athletes and environmental factors is crucial when designing and implementing effective talent management programmes. Comparing the results will allow refining current strategies and developing new approaches to talent management in speed skating.

5.2. Hypothesis testing

Overall, I believe that our hypothesis that **the players in the sport of short track speed skating are not unified in their understanding of the requirements of the sport, especially in the area of mental ability,** is supported by the results of the interviews and I will argue for this claim in this chapter.

According to the athletes, the cold environment, which is a fundamental element of speed skating, also poses a particular challenge that needs to be compensated by mental skills. The impact of cold temperatures on both muscle function and reaction time is significant. This is particularly important as athletes need to be in peak form in a short time, which requires fast and precise movements. Maintaining muscle tension and concentration in cold conditions a major challenge, which, according to Gatterer et al. (2021), requires continuous mental training on the part of athletes. Based on this research, it can be stated that speed skating conditions require considerable physical and mental adaptation and they need to maintain their performance despite the cold. The use of visualisation and other mental techniques not only improves physical performance, but also helps to prepare for competitive situations. The interviewees, including the sports psychologist, said that visualisation enables athletes to anticipate unexpected situations and mentally prepare for challenges on the track. This approach has proven to be particularly effective in short, high-intensity sports such as speed skating (Beauchamp et al., 2012). The coach highlighted that athletes often have only a few seconds to adapt to unexpected situations and make quick decisions. "In competition, every second counts and there is no time to rethink moves or hesitate," said the coach, suggesting that speed and concentration are essential for success. This observation is supported by McMorris and Rayment's (2007) research, which showed that during high-intensity, short-duration sporting activities, athletes' mental performance plays a key role in their success. According to athletes, the short, intense phases of speed skating competitions, where every move and decision is crucial, encourage them to develop mental resilience and the ability to cope with pressure. Mental preparation, such as concentration, stress management and the ability to react quickly, is essential to achieve high performance. In this respect, the study of gender differences is of particular importance. Interviews revealed that female athletes are often under greater pressure to meet expectations and often have different need more mental health support than their male counterparts. For female athletes, emotional support techniques are often more prevalent, while for men, competitive and results-focused approaches predominate. Coaches and sports psychologists have an important role to play in recognising and addressing this difference in mental training and tailoring their coaching methods to the needs of different genders of athletes. Taking into account individual needs, especially in the context of mental preparation, will enhance athletes' performance and help them to better manage the psychological stress associated with competition. This is a fundamental part of our hypothesis that short track speed skaters are not uniform in terms of the demands of the sport and mental preparation. The data collected in this study support the hypothesis that mental skills and their developmental methods may vary significantly between athletes, requiring further specific interventions in talent management strategies.

5.3. Practical suggestions

The following practical suggestions could be considered for the mental preparation of athletes, which are discussed in more detail in this chapter:

1. Personalised mental coaching
2. Stress management techniques
3. Developing communication skills
4. Non-specific training
5. Psychological support and family involvement

Short track speed skating is a mentally and physically demanding sport, where the development of mental skills is key to optimising athletes' performance. Below I detail practical suggestions that can support athletes, coaches and support staff in their mental preparation. Personalised mental preparation is an essential part of an athlete's success. Every athlete is unique, so taking into account the differences between the mental needs of men and women is essential. Sport psychologists play an important role in this process by helping to develop techniques that best suit the personality and mental needs of each athlete. The support provided by psychologists is critical not only in the pre-competitive period but also in maintaining long-term mental health.

Stress management techniques, such as relaxation exercises, breath control and meditation, help athletes to cope with the pressures of competition. Sports in cold environments are particularly challenging for athletes, so the use of stress management techniques is key to optimising mental and physical performance. Developing communication skills will further strengthen the relationship between athlete and coach. Open and honest communication helps athletes to share their feelings and fears with their coach, allowing coaches to provide more personalised support. Integrating communication training into training programmes can increase the effectiveness of teamwork and improve athlete performance. Last but not least, the involvement of family and immediate support circle in the mental preparation of athletes can increase emotional stability and mental health. Family support is of particular importance for young athletes, where the support of parents and other family members can help young people to better manage the stress of competition and training. By taking these practical suggestions into account and applying them appropriately, those involved in the sport of short track speed skating can deal more effectively with mental challenges, which can contribute to the long-term success of athletes and the development of the sport.

5.4. Further research opportunities

Current research has shown the impact on the development of mental skills in short track speed skaters and its impact on sport performance. Based on the results of this research, a number of further research directions have emerged, which could include a deeper analysis of different groups of athletes and further investigation of the effectiveness of training methods and mental support techniques. Areas where there is potential for further research are detailed below. One important area could be further investigation of gender differences. Although in our present research we have already touched on the differences between male and female athletes in the development of mental skills, a larger sample of specifically focused studies may be needed to analyse in more detail the effectiveness of different gender-specific training programmes and the development of athletes' mental health. In addition, the impact of mental skills development at different stages of athletes' careers would also be worth investigating. Research ranging from junior to experienced athletes could help to better understand at which age and with which methods the greatest improvements can be achieved. By developing and comparing programmes tailored to athletes of different ages, we can further training strategies can be refined. Further exploration of the role of family and social support may also be of particular importance. The present research has already highlighted the importance of family background, but the extent and nature of family and community support may vary in different cultural and social contexts. Comparing data from different countries may allow for more effective international programmes to be developed. Further analysis of coaching strategies and methods could also be an area of interest. Comparison of the different psychological and physical methods used by coaches, with a particular focus on technological innovations and new training tools, can help to develop the sport and improve the performance of competitors. Finally, the integration of the latest findings in sport psychology and cognitive sciences into speed skating training programmes could open up new perspectives. The application of neuropsychological studies and research focusing on cognitive development to the training and preparation of athletes will allow for a refinement of training methods on a scientific basis.

6.   Bibliography

Baker, J., Schorer, J., & Wattie, N. (2017).   Talent   In
                          Quest, 70(1),   48-
63. https://doi.org/10.1080/00336297.2017.1333438

Beauchamp, M. K., Harvey, R. H., & Beauchamp, P. H. (2012). An Integrated Biofeedback and Psychological Skills Training Program for Canada's Olympic Short-Track Speedskating Team. Journal of Clinical Sport Psychology, 6(1), 67-84. doi:10.1123/jcsp.6.1.67.

Bognár J., Trzaskoma-Bicsérdy G., Révész L., & Géczi G. (2006). The role of parents in sports talent management. Kalokagathia,1-2, pp. 86-96.

Boncz, I. (ed.) (2015). University of Pécs.

Burke, S., Sharp, L., Woods, D., & Paradis, K. F. (2021). Enhancing parental support through parent-education programs in youth sport: a systematic review. International Review of Sport and Exercise Psychology, 17(1), 208-235. https://doi.org/10.1080/1750984x.2021.1992793

Castellani, J. W., & Tipton, M. J. (2015).   Performance.   Comprehensive
                      Psychology,   6,   443–469.
https://doi.org/10.1002/cphy.c140081

Castellani, J. W., & Young, A. J. (2016). Human physiological responses to cold exposure: Acute responses and acclimatization to prolonged exposure. Autonomic Neuroscience, 196, 63-74. doi:10.1016/j.autneu.2016.02.009

Chapman, R. F., Stickford, J. L., & Levine, B. D. (2010). altitude training considerations for the winter sport athlete. Experimental Physiology, 95(3), 411-421. doi:10.1113/expphysiol.2009.050377

Cheung, S. S., Lee, J. K. W., & Oksa, J. (2016). thermal stress, human performance, and physical employment standards. applied physiology, nutrition, and metabolism, 41(6 (Suppl. 2)), S148-S164. doi:10.1139/apnm-2015-0518

Felser, S., Behrens, M., Fischer, S., Heise, S., Bäumler, M., Salomon, R., & Bruhn, S. (2015). Relationship between strength qualities and short track speed skating performance in young athletes. Scandinavian Journal of Medicine & Science in Sports, 26(2), 165-171. doi:10.1111/sms.12429

Gatterer, H., Dünnwald, T., Turner, R., Csapo, R., Schobersberger, W., Burtscher, M., Faulhaber, M., & Kennedy, M. D. (2021). Practicing Sport in Cold Environments: Practical Recommendations to Improve Sport Performance and Reduce Negative Health Outcomes. International Journal of Environmental Research and Public Health, 18(18), 9700. https://doi.org/10.3390/ijerph18189700.

Grainger, A., Kelly, A. L., Garland, S. W., Baker, J., Johnston, K., & McAuley, A. B. T. (2024). 'Athletes', 'Talents', and 'Players': Conceptual Distinctions and Considerations for Researchers and Practitioners. Sports Medicine. https://doi.org/10.1007/s40279-024-02101-5

Grant, A. M. (2006). A personal perspective on professional coaching and the development of coaching psychology. International Coaching Psychology Review, 1(1), 12-22. https://doi.org/10.53841/bpsicpr.2006.1.1.12

Grant, A. M., & Palmer, S. (2015). Invited Paper Integrating positive psychology and coaching psychology into counselling psychology. Counselling Psychology Review, 30(3), 22-25. https://doi.org/10.53841/bpscpr.2015.30.3.22

Griffo, J. M., Jensen, M., Anthony, C. C., Baghurst, T., & Kulinna, P. H. (2019). A decade of research literature in sport coaching (2005-2015). International Journal of Sports Science & Coaching, 174795411882505. doi:10.1177/1747954118825058

B. Kállay (2008). In Herczeg J. (ed.): J. (in Hungarian). Palatia Nyomda és Kiadó Kft., Sopron, 98-110.

Knight, C. J., Berrow, S. R., & Harwood, C. G. (2017). parenting in sport. Current Opinion in Psychology, 16, 93-97. doi:10.1016/j.copsyc.2017.03.011

Konings, M. J., Elferink-Gemser, M. T., Stoter, I. K., Van Der Meer, D., Otten, E., & Hettinga, F. J. (2014). Performance Characteristics of Long-Track Speed Skaters: A Literature Review. Sports Medicine, 45(4), 505-516. https://doi.org/10.1007/s40279-014-0298-z

Kuper, G.H., & Sterken, E. (2003). Endurance in speed skating: the development of world records. European Journal of Operational Research, 148(2), 293-301. doi:10.1016/s0377-2217(02)00685-9

McMorris, T., & Rayment, T. (2007). Short-Duration, High-Intensity Exercise and Performance of a Sports-Specific Skill: A Preliminary Study. Perceptual and Motor Skills, 105(2), 523-530. doi:10.2466/pms.105.2.523-530

Menting, S. G. P., Huijgen, B. C., Konings, M. J., Hettinga, F. J., & Elferink-Gemser, M. T. (2019). Pacing Behavior Development of Youth Short-Track Speed Skaters: A Longitudinal

Study. Medicine & Science in Sports & Exercise, 52(5), 1099-1108. https://doi.org/10.1249/mss.0000000000002239

Morrison, P., Pearsall, D. J., Turcotte, R. A., Lockwood, K., & Montgomery, D. L. (2005). skate blade hollow and oxygen consumption during forward skating. sports Engineering, 8(2), 91-
97. doi:10.1007/bf02844007

Nam, J., Choi, B., & Cho, E. (2022). exploring and developing a scale using item response theory for sport psychological skills in speed skaters. International Journal of Environmental Research and Public Health, 19(13), 8035. https://doi.org/10.3390/ijerph19138035

Noordhof, D. A., Mulder, R. C. M., de Koning, J. J., & Hopkins, W. G. (2016). race factors affecting performance times in elite long-track speed skating. international journal of sports physiology and performance, 11(4), 535-542. doi:10.1123/ijspp.2015-0171.

Oliver, A., McCarthy, P. J., & Burns, L. (2020). Teaching Athletes to Understand Their Attention Is Teaching Them to Concentrate. journal of sport psychology in action, 1-15. doi:10.1080/21520704.2020.1838980

Qurban, H., Wang, J., Siddique, H., Morris, T., & Qiao, Z. (2018). The mediating role of parental support: the relation between sports participation, self-esteem, and motivation for sports among Chinese students. current psychology, 38(2), 308-319. doi:10.1007/s12144-018-0016-3.

Renzulli, J. S. (1978) The nature of giftedness, In W. B. Barbe & J. S. Renzulli (Eds.), *The gifted and talented: Their education and development* (pp. 2-27). Columbus, OH: Merrill.

Telegdi, A. (2021). Innovation opportunities in the Hungarian speed skating methodology: the possibilities of adapting the long-term athlete preparation model in the Hungarian speed skating sports. Acta Universitatis de Carolo Eszterházy Nominatae. Sectio Sport (48). pp. 7-20. ISSN 26770105

Telegdi, A. (2023). The perception of the role of the coach the players of the Hungarian speed skating sport, In. Medovarszki, I. (Ed.) Subject-Pedagogical Kaleidoscope. Líceum Publishing House, Eger, pp. 141-154.

Telegdi, A.; Bognár, J. & Géczi, G. (2024). The role of the environment in speed skating talent management. 10.13140/RG.2.2.18129.85606.

Vaeyens, R., Lenoir, M., Williams, A. M., & Philippaerts, R. M. (2008). Talent Identification and Development Programmes in Sport. *Sports Medicine, 38*(9), 703- 714. https://doi.org/10.2165/00007256-200838090-00001

Wilks, B. (1991) Stress Management for Athletes. Sports Medicine, 11(5), 289-299. doi:10.2165/00007256-199111050-00002

Yang, Z., Ke, P., Zhang, Y., Du, F., & Hong, P. (2024). Quantitative analysis of the dominant external factors influencing elite speed skaters' performance using BP neural network. Frontiers in Sports and Active Living, 6. https://doi.org/10.3389/fspor.2024.1227785

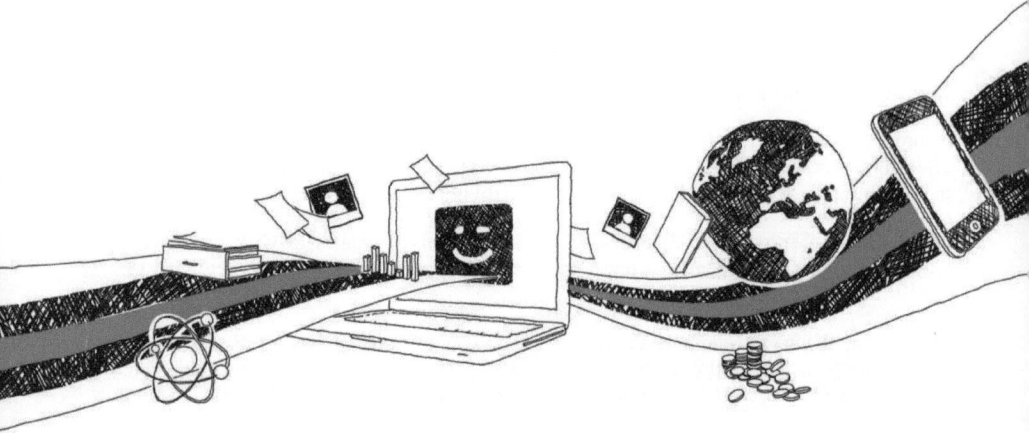
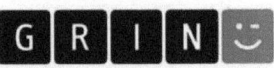